ENDOMORPH DIET

MAIN COURSE - 60+ Breakfast, Lunch, Dinner and Dessert Recipes for Endomorph Diet

TABLE OF CONTENTS

BREAKFAST 7
BLUEBERRY PANCAKES 7
ARTICHOKE PANCAKES 9
BANANA PANCAKES 10
KIWI PANCAKES 12
MELON PANCAKES 13
PRUNES MUFFINS 14
BANANA MUFFINS 16
CHERRY MUFFINS 18
STRAWBERRY MUFFINS 20
COCONUT MUFFINS 22
CARROT MUFFINS 24
ASIAN GREENS OMELETTE 26
BEANS OMELETTE 28
CABBAGE OMELETTE 30
MUSHROOM OMELETTE 32
TOMATO OMELETTE 34
OATS WITH PEANUT BUTTER 36
LUNCH 38
EGGS BENEDICT WITH HOLLANDAISE SAUCE 38
BAKED TOMATOES 40
MAPLE BACON 42
POTATO SALAD 43
LEBANESE BEAN SALAD 44
KALE & FENNEL SALAD 45

TOMATO & SPINACH SALAD	46
WILD RICE SALAD	47
KALE SALAD	48
THAI MANGO SALAD	49
HERBED SALAD	50
BEET SALAD	51
PEPITAS AND CRANBERRIES SALAD	52
OKRA FRITATTA	53
LEEK FRITATTA	55
KALE FRITATTA	57
GREENS FRITATTA	59
BROCCOLI FRITATTA	61
PESTO PASTA WITH ASPARAGUS	63
RICE NOODLES	64
EGG SANDWICH	66
CAULIFLOWER POPCORN	68
ROASTED CAULIFLOWER WITH ORANGE DRESSING	70
SIMPLE PIZZA RECIPE	72
ZUCCHINI PIZZA	73
DINNER	75
CAULIFLOWER RECIPE	75
BROCCOLI RECIPE	77
HAM PIZZA	78
CAULIFLOWER SOUP	80
ZUCCHINI SOUP	82
CELERY SOUP	84

CARROT SOUP 86

CUCUMBER SOUP 88

SMOOTHIES 91

TURMERIC-MANGO SMOOTHIE 91

AVOCADO-KALE SMOOTHIE 92

BUTTERMILK SMOOTHIE 93

GREEN SMOOTHIE 94

FRUIT SMOOTHIE 95

MANGO SMOOTHIE 96

DREAMSICLE SMOOTHIE 97

FIG SMOOTHIE 98

POMEGRANATE SMOOTHIE 99

GINGER-KALE SMOOTHIE 100

Copyright 2019 by Noah Jerris - All rights reserved.

This document is geared towards providing exact and reliable information in regards to the topic and issue covered. The publication is sold with the idea that the publisher is not required to render accounting, officially permitted, or otherwise, qualified services. If advice is necessary, legal or professional, a practiced individual in the profession should be ordered.

- From a Declaration of Principles which was accepted and approved equally by a Committee of the American Bar Association and a Committee of Publishers and Associations.

In no way is it legal to reproduce, duplicate, or transmit any part of this document in either electronic means or in printed format. Recording of this publication is strictly prohibited and any storage of this document is not allowed unless with written permission from the publisher. All rights reserved.

The information provided herein is stated to be truthful and consistent, in that any liability, in terms of inattention or otherwise, by any usage or abuse of any policies, processes, or directions contained within is the solitary and utter responsibility of the recipient reader. Under no circumstances will any legal responsibility or blame be held against the publisher for any reparation, damages, or monetary loss due to the information herein, either directly or indirectly.

Respective authors own all copyrights not held by the publisher.

The information herein is offered for informational

purposes solely, and is universal as so. The presentation of the information is without contract or any type of guarantee assurance.

The trademarks that are used are without any consent, and the publication of the trademark is without permission or backing by the trademark owner. All trademarks and brands within this book are for clarifying purposes only and are the owned by the owners themselves, not affiliated with this document.

Introduction

Endomorph recipes for personal enjoyment but also for family enjoyment. You will love them for sure for how easy it is to prepare them.

BREAKFAST

BLUEBERRY PANCAKES

Serves: **4**
Prep Time: **10** Minutes
Cook Time: **20** Minutes
Total Time: **30** Minutes

INGREDIENTS

- 1 cup whole wheat flour
- ¼ tsp baking soda
- ¼ tsp baking powder
- 1 cup blueberries
- 2 eggs
- 1 cup milk

DIRECTIONS

1. In a bowl combine all ingredients together and mix well
2. In a skillet heat olive oil

3. Pour ¼ of the batter and cook each pancake for 1-2 minutes per side
4. When ready remove from heat and serve

ARTICHOKE PANCAKES

Serves: **4**
Prep Time: **10** Minutes
Cook Time: **30** Minutes
Total Time: **40** Minutes

INGREDIENTS

- 1 cup whole wheat flour
- ¼ tsp baking soda
- ¼ tsp baking powder
- 1 cup artichoke
- 2 eggs
- 1 cup milk

DIRECTIONS

1. In a bowl combine all ingredients together and mix well
2. In a skillet heat olive oil
3. Pour ¼ of the batter and cook each pancake for 1-2 minutes per side
4. When ready remove from heat and serve

BANANA PANCAKES

Serves: **4**

Prep Time: **10** Minutes

Cook Time: **20** Minutes

Total Time: **30** Minutes

INGREDIENTS

- 1 cup whole wheat flour
- ¼ tsp baking soda
- ¼ tsp baking powder
- 1 cup mashed banana
- 2 eggs
- 1 cup milk
-

DIRECTIONS

1. In a bowl combine all ingredients together and mix well
2. In a skillet heat olive oil
3. Pour ¼ of the batter and cook each pancake for 1-2 minutes per side

4. When ready remove from heat and serve

KIWI PANCAKES

Serves: **4**

Prep Time: **10** Minutes

Cook Time: **20** Minutes

Total Time: **30** Minutes

INGREDIENTS

- 1 cup whole wheat flour
- ¼ tsp baking soda
- ¼ tsp baking powder
- 1 cup kiwi
- 2 eggs
- 1 cup milk

DIRECTIONS

1. In a bowl combine all ingredients together and mix well
2. In a skillet heat olive oil
3. Pour ¼ of the batter and cook each pancake for 1-2 minutes per side
4. When ready remove from heat and serve

MELON PANCAKES

Serves: **4**

Prep Time: **10** Minutes

Cook Time: **30** Minutes

Total Time: **40** Minutes

INGREDIENTS

- 1 cup whole wheat flour
- ¼ tsp baking soda
- ¼ tsp baking powder
- 2 eggs
- 1 cup mashed melon
- 1 cup milk

DIRECTIONS

1. In a bowl combine all ingredients together and mix well
2. In a skillet heat olive oil
3. Pour ¼ of the batter and cook each pancake for 1-2 minutes per side
4. When ready remove from heat and serve

PRUNES MUFFINS

Serves: **8-12**

Prep Time: **10** Minutes

Cook Time: **20** Minutes

Total Time: **30** Minutes

INGREDIENTS

- 2 eggs
- 1 tablespoon olive oil
- 1 cup milk
- 2 cups whole wheat flour
- 1 tsp baking soda
- ¼ tsp baking soda
- 1 tsp ginger
- 1 cup prunes
- ¼ cup molasses

DIRECTIONS

1. In a bowl combine all dry ingredients
2. In another bowl combine all dry ingredients

3. Combine wet and dry ingredients together
4. Pour mixture into 8-12 prepared muffin cups, fill 2/3 of the cups
5. Bake for 18-20 minutes at 375 F
6. When ready remove from the oven and serve

BANANA MUFFINS

Serves: **8-12**

Prep Time: **10** Minutes

Cook Time: **20** Minutes

Total Time: **30** Minutes

INGREDIENTS

- 2 eggs
- 1 tablespoon olive oil
- 1 cup milk
- 2 cups whole wheat flour
- 1 tsp baking soda
- ¼ tsp baking soda
- 1 tsp cinnamon
- 1 cup mashed banana

DIRECTIONS

1. In a bowl combine all dry ingredients
2. In another bowl combine all dry ingredients
3. Combine wet and dry ingredients together

4. Fold in mashed banana and mix well
5. Pour mixture into 8-12 prepared muffin cups, fill 2/3 of the cups
6. Bake for 18-20 minutes at 375 F
7. When ready remove from the oven and serve

CHERRY MUFFINS

Serves: **8-12**

Prep Time: **10** Minutes

Cook Time: **20** Minutes

Total Time: **30** Minutes

INGREDIENTS

- 2 eggs
- 1 tablespoon olive oil
- 1 cup milk
- 2 cups whole wheat flour
- 1 tsp baking soda
- ¼ tsp baking soda
- 1 tsp cinnamon
- 1 cup cherries

DIRECTIONS

1. In a bowl combine all dry ingredients
2. In another bowl combine all dry ingredients
3. Combine wet and dry ingredients together

4. Fold in cherries and mix well
5. Pour mixture into 8-12 prepared muffin cups, fill 2/3 of the cups
6. Bake for 18-20 minutes at 375 F
7. When ready remove from the oven and serve

STRAWBERRY MUFFINS

Serves: **8-12**

Prep Time: **10** Minutes

Cook Time: **20** Minutes

Total Time: **30** Minutes

INGREDIENTS

- 2 eggs
- 1 tablespoon olive oil
- 1 cup milk
- 2 cups whole wheat flour
- 1 tsp baking soda
- ¼ tsp baking soda
- 1 tsp cinnamon
- 1 cup strawberries

DIRECTIONS

1. In a bowl combine all dry ingredients
2. In another bowl combine all dry ingredients
3. Combine wet and dry ingredients together

4. Fold in strawberries and mix well
5. Pour mixture into 8-12 prepared muffin cups, fill 2/3 of the cups
6. Bake for 18-20 minutes at 375 F
7. When ready remove from the oven and serve

COCONUT MUFFINS

Serves: **8-12**

Prep Time: **10** Minutes

Cook Time: **20** Minutes

Total Time: **30** Minutes

INGREDIENTS

- 2 eggs
- 1 tablespoon olive oil
- 1 cup milk
- 2 cups whole wheat flour
- 1 tsp baking soda
- ¼ tsp baking soda
- 1 tsp cinnamon
- 1 cup coconut flakes

DIRECTIONS

1. In a bowl combine all dry ingredients
2. In another bowl combine all dry ingredients
3. Combine wet and dry ingredients together

4. Pour mixture into 8-12 prepared muffin cups, fill 2/3 of the cups
5. Bake for 18-20 minutes at 375 F
6. When ready remove from the oven and serve

CARROT MUFFINS

Serves: **8-12**

Prep Time: **10** Minutes

Cook Time: **20** Minutes

Total Time: **30** Minutes

INGREDIENTS

- 2 eggs
- 1 tablespoon olive oil
- 1 cup milk
- 2 cups whole wheat flour
- 1 tsp baking soda
- ¼ tsp baking soda
- 1 cut carrot
- 1 tsp cinnamon

DIRECTIONS

1. In a bowl combine all dry ingredients
2. In another bowl combine all dry ingredients
3. Combine wet and dry ingredients together

4. Pour mixture into 8-12 prepared muffin cups, fill 2/3 of the cups
5. Bake for 18-20 minutes at 375 F
6. When ready remove from the oven and serve

ASIAN GREENS OMELETTE

Serves: *1*
Prep Time: *5* Minutes
Cook Time: *10* Minutes
Total Time: *15* Minutes

INGREDIENTS

- 2 eggs
- ¼ tsp salt
- ¼ tsp black pepper
- 1 tablespoon olive oil
- ¼ cup cheese
- ¼ tsp basil
- 1 cup Asian greens

DIRECTIONS

1. In a bowl combine all ingredients together and mix well
2. In a skillet heat olive oil and pour the egg mixture
3. Cook for 1-2 minutes per side

4. When ready remove omelette from the skillet and serve

BEANS OMELETTE

Serves: **1**
Prep Time: **5** Minutes
Cook Time: **10** Minutes
Total Time: **15** Minutes

INGREDIENTS

- 2 eggs
- ¼ tsp salt
- ¼ tsp black pepper
- 1 tablespoon olive oil
- ¼ cup cheese
- ¼ tsp basil
- 1 cup beans

DIRECTIONS

1. In a bowl combine all ingredients together and mix well
2. In a skillet heat olive oil and pour the egg mixture
3. Cook for 1-2 minutes per side

4. When ready remove omelette from the skillet and serve

CABBAGE OMELETTE

Serves: **1**

Prep Time: **5** Minutes

Cook Time: **10** Minutes

Total Time: **15** Minutes

INGREDIENTS

- 2 eggs
- ¼ tsp salt
- ¼ tsp black pepper
- 1 tablespoon olive oil
- ¼ cup cheese
- ¼ tsp basil
- 1 cup red onion
- 1 cup cabbage

DIRECTIONS

1. In a bowl combine all ingredients together and mix well
2. In a skillet heat olive oil and pour the egg mixture

3. Cook for 1-2 minutes per side
4. When ready remove omelette from the skillet and serve

MUSHROOM OMELETTE

Serves: *1*

Prep Time: *5* Minutes

Cook Time: *10* Minutes

Total Time: *15* Minutes

INGREDIENTS

- 2 eggs
- ¼ tsp salt
- ¼ tsp black pepper
- 1 tablespoon olive oil
- ¼ cup cheese
- ¼ tsp basil
- 1 cup mushrooms

DIRECTIONS

1. In a bowl combine all ingredients together and mix well
2. In a skillet heat olive oil and pour the egg mixture
3. Cook for 1-2 minutes per side

4. When ready remove omelette from the skillet and serve

TOMATO OMELETTE

Serves: **1**

Prep Time: **5** Minutes

Cook Time: **10** Minutes

Total Time: **15** Minutes

INGREDIENTS

- 2 eggs
- ¼ tsp salt
- ¼ tsp black pepper
- 1 tablespoon olive oil
- ¼ cup cheese
- ¼ tsp basil
- 1 cup tomatoes

DIRECTIONS

1. In a bowl combine all ingredients together and mix well
2. In a skillet heat olive oil and pour the egg mixture
3. Cook for 1-2 minutes per side

4. When ready remove omelette from the skillet and serve

OATS WITH PEANUT BUTTER

Serves: **1**

Prep Time: **5** Minutes

Cook Time: **5** Minutes

Total Time: **10** Minutes

INGREDIENTS

- 1 cup oats
- 3 tablespoons peanut butter
- ½ cup almond milk
- ¼ banana

DIRECTIONS

1. **In a bowl combine all ingredients together and mix well**
2. **Pour mixture into a jar**
3. **Refrigerate overnight**
4. **Serve in the morning**

LUNCH

EGGS BENEDICT WITH HOLLANDAISE SAUCE

Serves: **2**

Prep Time: **10** Minutes

Cook Time: **15** Minutes

Total Time: **25** Minutes

INGREDIENTS

- 4 English muffins
- 4 poached eggs
- 4 slices ham
- 2 tsp butter
- 1 cup Hollandaise sauce

DIRECTIONS

1. Cut English muffins in half
2. Spread butter on each muffin half
3. Top each muffin with ham and poached eggs
4. Add 2-3 tablespoons of hollandaise sauce on each muffin

5. Serve when ready

BAKED TOMATOES

Serves: **4**

Prep Time: **10** Minutes

Cook Time: **20** Minutes

Total Time: **30** Minutes

INGREDIENTS

- 2-3 tablespoons olive oil
- 4 eggs
- ¼ cup parmesan cheese
- 4 tomatoes
- 1 tsp herbs
- 1 tsp parsley
- ¼ tsp salt

DIRECTIONS

1. Cut the stems of the tomatoes and remove them
2. Scoop out the interior of the tomatoes
3. Crack an egg into each tomato

4. Top with parmesan cheese, herbs, parsley and salt
5. Bake at 400 F for 18-20 minutes
6. When ready remove from the oven and serve

MAPLE BACON

Serves: **4**

Prep Time: **5** Minutes

Cook Time: **15** Minutes

Total Time: **20** Minutes

INGREDIENTS

- 1 lb. bacon
- ¼ cup sugar
- ½ cup maple syrup

DIRECTIONS

1. Place the bacon on a baking sheet
2. Brush the bacon with maple syrup and sprinkle with sugar
3. Bake at 400 F for 12-15 minutes or until crispy
4. When ready remove from the oven and serve

POTATO SALAD

Serves: 2
Prep Time: 5 Minutes
Cook Time: 5 Minutes
Total Time: 10 Minutes

INGREDIENTS

- 2 lb. cooked red potatoes
- 1 tablespoon salt
- ¼ cup olive oil
- ¼ cup parsley
- ¼ cup green onions
- 1 tablespoon lemon juice
- 1 tsp mustard
- 2 stalks celery

DIRECTIONS

1. In a bowl mix all ingredients and mix well
2. Serve with dressing

LEBANESE BEAN SALAD

Serves: 2
Prep Time: 5 Minutes
Cook Time: 5 Minutes
Total Time: 10 Minutes

INGREDIENTS

- 1 can black beans
- 1 can chickpeas
- 1 red onion
- 2 stalks celery
- 1 cucumber
- ½ cup parsley
- 1 tablespoon mint
- 2 cloves garlic

DIRECTIONS

1. In a bowl mix all ingredients and mix well
2. Serve with dressing

KALE & FENNEL SALAD

Serves: **2**

Prep Time: **5** Minutes

Cook Time: **5** Minutes

Total Time: **10** Minutes

INGREDIENTS

- 1 bunch kale
- 1 apple
- 1 fennel
- 4 oz. feta cheese
- ½ cup cranberries
- 1 cup maple syrup salad dressing

DIRECTIONS

1. **In a bowl mix all ingredients and mix well**
2. **Serve with dressing**

TOMATO & SPINACH SALAD

Serves: 2
Prep Time: 5 Minutes
Cook Time: 5 Minutes
Total Time: 10 Minutes

INGREDIENTS

- 1 cup quinoa
- 1 cup tomatoes
- 1 cup baby spinach
- 1 tablespoon olive oil
- 1 cup lemon salad dressing

DIRECTIONS

1. In a bowl mix all ingredients and mix well
2. Serve with dressing

WILD RICE SALAD

Serves: **2**

Prep Time: **5** Minutes

Cook Time: **5** Minutes

Total Time: **10** Minutes

INGREDIENTS

- 1 cup cooked wild rice
- 1 tsp olive oil
- 6 oz. arugula
- ¼ cup basil
- ½ cup cranberries
- ½ cup goat cheese
- 1 cup lemon salad dressing

DIRECTIONS

1. In a bowl mix all ingredients and mix well
2. Serve with dressing

KALE SALAD

Serves: **2**

Prep Time: **5** Minutes

Cook Time: **5** Minutes

Total Time: **10** Minutes

INGREDIENTS

- 1 bunch kale
- 1 cup cooked grains
- 2 carrots
- 1 radish
- 1 tablespoon pepitas
- 1 cup tahini dressing

DIRECTIONS

1. In a bowl mix all ingredients and mix well
2. Serve with dressing

THAI MANGO SALAD

Serves: 2
Prep Time: 5 Minutes
Cook Time: 5 Minutes
Total Time: 10 Minutes

INGREDIENTS

- 1 head leaf lettuce
- 1 red bell pepper
- 2 mangoes
- 1 cup green onion
- ½ cup peanuts
- ½ cup cilantro
- 1 cup peanut dressing

DIRECTIONS

1. In a bowl mix all ingredients and mix well
2. Serve with dressing

HERBED SALAD

Serves: 2

Prep Time: 5 Minutes

Cook Time: 5 Minutes

Total Time: 10 Minutes

INGREDIENTS

- 2 lb. cooked white potatoes
- 2 tablespoons olive oil
- ½ cup parsley
- ½ cup green onion
- 1 tablespoon lemon juice
- 1 tsp mustard
- 2 cloves garlic
- 1 tsp black pepper
- 1 tsp oregano

DIRECTIONS

1. In a bowl mix all ingredients and mix well
2. Serve with dressing

BEET SALAD

Serves: **2**

Prep Time: **5** Minutes

Cook Time: **5** Minutes

Total Time: **10** Minutes

INGREDIENTS

- 1 cup cooked quinoa
- 1 cup edamame
- 1 cup pepitas
- 1 beet
- 1 carrot
- 1 cup baby spinach
- 1 avocado
- 1 cup lemon salad dressing

DIRECTIONS

1. **In a bowl mix all ingredients and mix well**
2. **Serve with dressing**

PEPITAS AND CRANBERRIES SALAD

Serves: 2
Prep Time: 5 Minutes
Cook Time: 5 Minutes
Total Time: 10 Minutes

INGREDIENTS

- 6 oz. greens
- 1 apple
- 1 cup cranberries
- ½ cup pepitas
- 3 oz. feta cheese

DIRECTIONS

1. In a bowl mix all ingredients and mix well
2. Serve with dressing

OKRA FRITATTA

Serves: **2**

Prep Time: **10** Minutes

Cook Time: **20** Minutes

Total Time: **30** Minutes

INGREDIENTS

- ½ lb. okra
- 1 tablespoon olive oil
- ½ red onion
- 2 eggs
- ¼ tsp salt
- 2 oz. cheddar cheese
- 1 garlic clove
- ¼ tsp dill

DIRECTIONS

1. In a bowl whisk eggs with salt and cheese
2. In a frying pan heat olive oil and pour egg mixture

3. Add remaining ingredients and mix well
4. Serve when ready

LEEK FRITATTA

Serves: 2
Prep Time: 10 Minutes
Cook Time: 20 Minutes
Total Time: 30 Minutes

INGREDIENTS

- ½ lb. leek
- 1 tablespoon olive oil
- ½ red onion
- ¼ tsp salt
- 2 ggs
- 2 oz. cheddar cheese
- 1 garlic clove
- ¼ tsp dill

DIRECTIONS

1. In a bowl whisk eggs with salt and cheese
2. In a frying pan heat olive oil and pour egg mixture

3. Add remaining ingredients and mix well
4. Serve when ready

KALE FRITATTA

Serves: 2

Prep Time: 10 Minutes

Cook Time: 20 Minutes

Total Time: 30 Minutes

INGREDIENTS

- 1 cup kale
- 1 tablespoon olive oil
- ½ red onion
- ¼ tsp salt
- 2 eggs
- 2 oz. cheddar cheese
- 1 garlic clove
- ¼ tsp dill

DIRECTIONS

1. In a skillet sauté kale until tender
2. In a bowl whisk eggs with salt and cheese

3. In a frying pan heat olive oil and pour egg mixture
4. Add remaining ingredients and mix well
5. Serve when ready

GREENS FRITATTA

Serves: **2**

Prep Time: **10** Minutes

Cook Time: **20** Minutes

Total Time: **30** Minutes

INGREDIENTS

- ½ lb. greens
- 1 tablespoon olive oil
- ½ red onion
- ¼ tsp salt
- 2 eggs
- 2 oz. parmesan cheese
- 1 garlic clove
- ¼ tsp dill

DIRECTIONS

1. In a bowl whisk eggs with salt and parmesan cheese
2. In a frying pan heat olive oil and pour egg mixture

3. Add remaining ingredients and mix well
4. Serve when ready

BROCCOLI FRITATTA

Serves: **2**

Prep Time: **10** Minutes

Cook Time: **20** Minutes

Total Time: **30** Minutes

INGREDIENTS

- 1 cup broccoli
- 1 tablespoon olive oil
- ½ red onion
- ¼ tsp salt
- 2 oz. cheddar cheese
- 1 garlic clove
- ¼ tsp dill

DIRECTIONS

1. In a skillet sauté broccoli until tender
2. In a bowl whisk eggs with salt and cheese
3. In a frying pan heat olive oil and pour egg mixture

4. Add remaining ingredients and mix well
5. When ready serve with sautéed broccoli

PESTO PASTA WITH ASPARAGUS

Serves: **4**
Prep Time: **10** Minutes
Cook Time: **20** Minutes
Total Time: **30** Minutes

INGREDIENTS

- 10 oz. shell pasta
- 1 lb. asparagus
- 2-3 tablespoons olive oil
- ¼ cup basil pesto
- ½ cup dried tomatoes
- ½ cup mozzarella cheese

DIRECTIONS

1. In a pot boil water and cook pasta
2. Place asparagus on a baking sheet drizzle olive oil and bake at 400 F for 12-15 minutes
3. In a bowl combine roasted asparagus, pasta, pesto and dried tomatoes
4. Top with mozzarella cheese and serve

RICE NOODLES

Serves: 2

Prep Time: 10 Minutes

Cook Time: 20 Minutes

Total Time: 30 Minutes

INGREDIENTS

- 1 lb. rice noodles
- 2 tablespoons olive oil
- 1 red onion
- ½ lb. prawns
- 1 red pepper
- ¼ cucumber
- 1 tablespoon coriander leaves
- 3 tablespoon soy sauce
- 2 tablespoons fish sauce

DIRECTIONS

1. **In a bowl combine soy sauce and fish sauce together**

2. In a skillet heat olive oil and sauté onion until soft
3. Add prawns and sauce mixture to the skillet
4. Remove from heat, add pasta and remaining ingredients
5. Mix well and serve

EGG SANDWICH

Serves: **4**

Prep Time: **10** Minutes

Cook Time: **30** Minutes

Total Time: **40** Minutes

INGREDIENTS

- 1 lb. beetroot
- 2-3 bay leaves
- 2-3 eggs
- 2 tablespoons mayonnaise
- 2 celery sticks
- 1 pack mini peppers
- 1 gluten-free baton

DIRECTIONS

1. Slice the beetroot and fry for 2-3 minutes
2. Boil the eggs and cut in half
3. Cut the bread in half and spread mayonnaise on each bread half

4. Top with beetroot, bay leaves, celery sticks, peppers and boiled eggs
5. Serve when ready

CAULIFLOWER POPCORN

Serves: **4-6**

Prep Time: **10** Minutes

Cook Time: **25** Minutes

Total Time: **35** Minutes

INGREDIENTS

- 1 cauliflower
- 1 tsp cumin
- 1 tsp turmeric
- 1 tsp chilies
- 1 tsp olive oil

DIRECTIONS

1. Cut the cauliflower into small pieces
2. In a bowl combine cumin, turmeric and chilies together
3. Add the cauliflower to the mixture and toss to coat
4. Drizzle olive oil and roast at 400 F for 22-25 minutes

5. When crispy remove from the oven and serve

ROASTED CAULIFLOWER WITH ORANGE DRESSING

Serves: **4**

Prep Time: **10** Minutes

Cook Time: **30** Minutes

Total Time: **40** Minutes

INGREDIENTS

- 1 cauliflower
- 2 tablespoons olive oil
- 1 tsp cumin seeds
- 1 garlic clove
- 1 tsp chillies
- 1 tsp parsley
- Juice from 1 orange

DIRECTIONS

1. In a pan bring water to a boil and place the cauliflower
2. Simmer on medium heat for 5-10 minutes
3. In a bowl combine parsley, cumin seeds, chilies, olive oil and mix well

4. Toss the cauliflower florets with the mixture
5. Drizzle orange juice over the florets
6. Roast at 400 F for 18-20 minutes
7. When ready remove from the oven and serve

SIMPLE PIZZA RECIPE

Serves: **_6-8_**

Prep Time: **_10_** Minutes

Cook Time: **_15_** Minutes

Total Time: **_25_** Minutes

INGREDIENTS

- 1 pizza crust
- ½ cup tomato sauce
- ¼ black pepper
- 1 cup pepperoni slices
- 1 cup mozzarella cheese
- 1 cup olives

DIRECTIONS

1. Spread tomato sauce on the pizza crust
2. Place all the toppings on the pizza crust
3. Bake the pizza at 425 F for 12-15 minutes
4. When ready remove pizza from the oven and serve

ZUCCHINI PIZZA

Serves: **6-8**
Prep Time: **10** Minutes
Cook Time: **15** Minutes
Total Time: **25** Minutes

INGREDIENTS

- 1 pizza crust
- ½ cup tomato sauce
- ¼ black pepper
- 1 cup zucchini slices
- 1 cup mozzarella cheese
- 1 cup olives

DIRECTIONS

1. Spread tomato sauce on the pizza crust
2. Place all the toppings on the pizza crust
3. Bake the pizza at 425 F for 12-15 minutes
4. When ready remove pizza from the oven and serve

DINNER

CAULIFLOWER RECIPE

Serves: **6-8**
Prep Time: **10** Minutes
Cook Time: **15** Minutes
Total Time: **25** Minutes

INGREDIENTS

- 1 pizza crust
- ½ cup tomato sauce
- ¼ black pepper
- 1 cup cauliflower
- 1 cup mozzarella cheese
- 1 cup olives

DIRECTIONS

1. Spread tomato sauce on the pizza crust
2. Place all the toppings on the pizza crust
3. Bake the pizza at 425 F for 12-15 minutes

4. When ready remove pizza from the oven and serve

BROCCOLI RECIPE

Serves: **6-8**

Prep Time: **10** Minutes

Cook Time: **15** Minutes

Total Time: **25** Minutes

INGREDIENTS

- 1 pizza crust
- ½ cup tomato sauce
- ¼ black pepper
- 1 cup broccoli
- 1 cup mozzarella cheese
- 1 cup olives

DIRECTIONS

1. Spread tomato sauce on the pizza crust
2. Place all the toppings on the pizza crust
3. Bake the pizza at 425 F for 12-15 minutes
4. When ready remove pizza from the oven and serve

HAM PIZZA

Serves: **6-8**

Prep Time: **10** Minutes

Cook Time: **15** Minutes

Total Time: **25** Minutes

INGREDIENTS

- 1 pizza crust
- ½ cup tomato sauce
- ¼ black pepper
- 1 cup pepperoni slices
- 1 cup tomatoes
- 6-8 ham slices
- 1 cup mozzarella cheese
- 1 cup olives

DIRECTIONS

1. Spread tomato sauce on the pizza crust
2. Place all the toppings on the pizza crust
3. Bake the pizza at 425 F for 12-15 minutes

4. When ready remove pizza from the oven and serve

CAULIFLOWER SOUP

Serves: **4**

Prep Time: **10** Minutes

Cook Time: **20** Minutes

Total Time: **30** Minutes

INGREDIENTS

- 1 tablespoon olive oil
- 1 lb. cauliflower
- ¼ red onion
- ½ cup all-purpose flour
- ¼ tsp salt
- ¼ tsp pepper
- 1 can vegetable broth
- 1 cup heavy cream

DIRECTIONS

1. In a saucepan heat olive oil and sauté cauliflower until tender
2. Add remaining ingredients to the saucepan and bring to a boil

3. When all the vegetables are tender transfer to a blender and blend until smooth
4. Pour soup into bowls, garnish with parsley and serve

ZUCCHINI SOUP

Serves: **4**

Prep Time: **10** Minutes

Cook Time: **20** Minutes

Total Time: **30** Minutes

INGREDIENTS

- 1 tablespoon olive oil
- 1 lb. zucchini
- ¼ red onion
- ½ cup all-purpose flour
- ¼ tsp salt
- ¼ tsp pepper
- 1 can vegetable broth
- 1 cup heavy cream

DIRECTIONS

1. In a saucepan heat olive oil and sauté zucchini until tender
2. Add remaining ingredients to the saucepan and bring to a boil

3. When all the vegetables are tender transfer to a blender and blend until smooth
4. Pour soup into bowls, garnish with parsley and serve

CELERY SOUP

Serves: *4*

Prep Time: *10* Minutes

Cook Time: *20* Minutes

Total Time: *30* Minutes

INGREDIENTS

- 1 tablespoon olive oil
- 1 lb. celery
- ¼ red onion
- ½ cup all-purpose flour
- ¼ tsp salt
- ¼ tsp pepper
- 1 can vegetable broth
- 1 cup heavy cream

DIRECTIONS

1. In a saucepan heat olive oil and sauté celery until tender
2. Add remaining ingredients to the saucepan and bring to a boil

3. When all the vegetables are tender transfer to a blender and blend until smooth
4. Pour soup into bowls, garnish with parsley and serve

CARROT SOUP

Serves: **4**

Prep Time: **10** Minutes

Cook Time: **20** Minutes

Total Time: **30** Minutes

INGREDIENTS

- 1 tablespoon olive oil
- 1 lb. carrots
- ¼ red onion
- ½ cup all-purpose flour
- ¼ tsp salt
- ¼ tsp pepper
- 1 can vegetable broth
- 1 cup heavy cream

DIRECTIONS

1. In a saucepan heat olive oil and sauté carrots until tender
2. Add remaining ingredients to the saucepan and bring to a boil

3. When all the vegetables are tender transfer to a blender and blend until smooth
4. Pour soup into bowls, garnish with parsley and serve

CUCUMBER SOUP

Serves: **4**

Prep Time: **10** Minutes

Cook Time: **20** Minutes

Total Time: **30** Minutes

INGREDIENTS

- 1 tablespoon olive oil
- 1 lb. cucumber
- ¼ red onion
- ½ cup all-purpose flour
- ¼ tsp salt
- ¼ tsp pepper
- 1 can vegetable broth
- 1 cup heavy cream

DIRECTIONS

1. In a saucepan heat olive oil and sauté cucumber until tender
2. Add remaining ingredients to the saucepan and bring to a boil

3. When all the vegetables are tender transfer to a blender and blend until smooth
4. Pour soup into bowls, garnish with parsley and serve

SMOOTHIES

TURMERIC-MANGO SMOOTHIE

Serves: *1*
Prep Time: *5* Minutes
Cook Time: *5* Minutes
Total Time: *10* Minutes

INGREDIENTS

- 1 cup Greek yogurt
- ¼ cup orange juice
- 1 banana
- 1 tablespoon turmeric
- 1 tsp vanilla extract
- 1 cup ice

DIRECTIONS

1. **In a blender place all ingredients and blend until smooth**
2. **Pour smoothie in a glass and serve**

AVOCADO-KALE SMOOTHIE

Serves: **1**
Prep Time: **5** Minutes
Cook Time: **5** Minutes
Total Time: **10** Minutes

INGREDIENTS

- 1 cup coconut milk
- 1 tablespoon lemon juice
- 1 bunch kale
- 1 cup spinach
- ¼ avocado
- 1 cup ice

DIRECTIONS

1. In a blender place all ingredients and blend until smooth
2. Pour smoothie in a glass and serve

BUTTERMILK SMOOTHIE

Serves: *1*

Prep Time: *5* Minutes

Cook Time: *5* Minutes

Total Time: *10* Minutes

INGREDIENTS

- 1 cup ice
- 1 cup strawberries
- 1 cup blueberries
- 1 cup buttermilk
- ½ tsp vanilla extract

DIRECTIONS

1. **In a blender place all ingredients and blend until smooth**
2. **Pour smoothie in a glass and serve**

GREEN SMOOTHIE

Serves: **1**

Prep Time: **5** Minutes

Cook Time: **5** Minutes

Total Time: **10** Minutes

INGREDIENTS

- 1 cup berries
- 1 cup baby spinach
- 1 tablespoon orange juice
- ¼ cup coconut water
- ½ cup Greek yogurt

DIRECTIONS

1. **In a blender place all ingredients and blend until smooth**
2. **Pour smoothie in a glass and serve**

FRUIT SMOOTHIE

Serves: *1*

Prep Time: *5* Minutes

Cook Time: *5* Minutes

Total Time: *10* Minutes

INGREDIENTS

- 1 mango
- 1 cup vanilla yogurt
- 2 tablespoons honey
- 1 tablespoon lime juice
- 1 banana
- 1 can strawberries
- 1 kiwi

DIRECTIONS

1. In a blender place all ingredients and blend until smooth
2. Pour smoothie in a glass and serve

MANGO SMOOTHIE

Serves: **1**

Prep Time: **5** Minutes

Cook Time: **5** Minutes

Total Time: **10** Minutes

INGREDIENTS

- 2 cups mango
- 1 cup buttermilk
- 1 tsp vanilla extract
- 1 cup kiwi
- ½ cup coconut milk

DIRECTIONS

1. In a blender place all ingredients and blend until smooth
2. Pour smoothie in a glass and serve

DREAMSICLE SMOOTHIE

Serves: *1*
Prep Time: *5* Minutes
Cook Time: *5* Minutes
Total Time: *10* Minutes

INGREDIENTS

- 1 cup Greek yogurt
- 1 cup ice
- ¼ cup mango
- 1 orange
- 1 pinch cinnamon

DIRECTIONS

1. In a blender place all ingredients and blend until smooth
2. Pour smoothie in a glass and serve

FIG SMOOTHIE

Serves: **1**

Prep Time: **5** Minutes

Cook Time: **5** Minutes

Total Time: **10** Minutes

INGREDIENTS

- 1 cup ice
- 1 cup vanilla yogurt
- 1 cup coconut milk
- 1 tsp honey
- 4 figs

DIRECTIONS

1. In a blender place all ingredients and blend until smooth
2. Pour smoothie in a glass and serve

POMEGRANATE SMOOTHIE

Serves: *1*
Prep Time: *5* Minutes
Cook Time: *5* Minutes
Total Time: *10* Minutes

INGREDIENTS

- 2 cups blueberries
- 1 cup pomegranate
- 1 tablespoon honey
- 1 cup Greek yogurt

DIRECTIONS

1. **In a blender place all ingredients and blend until smooth**
2. **Pour smoothie in a glass and serve**

GINGER-KALE SMOOTHIE

Serves: *1*
Prep Time: *5* Minutes
Cook Time: *5* Minutes
Total Time: *10* Minutes

INGREDIENTS

- 1 cup kale
- 1 banana
- 1 cup almond milk
- 1 cup vanilla yogurt
- 1 tsp chia seeds
- ¼ tsp ginger

DIRECTIONS

1. In a blender place all ingredients and blend until smooth
2. Pour smoothie in a glass and serve

THANK YOU FOR READING THIS BOOK!

Made in the USA
Monee, IL
10 May 2022